The Vegetables Save The Farm

Written by: SHARIng Health with Shari

Illustrations by: Sherry Misso

ISBN-13: 978-1540555618
ISBN-10: 1540555615

Special thanks to all who went through the process of writing this book with me. Thank you Christopher for not thinking I was crazy when I said, "I'm going to write a book." Thanks to those who did edits for me and gave me feedback. Special thanks to Sherry Misso for bringing my vegetables to life, I am grateful the universe brought us together.

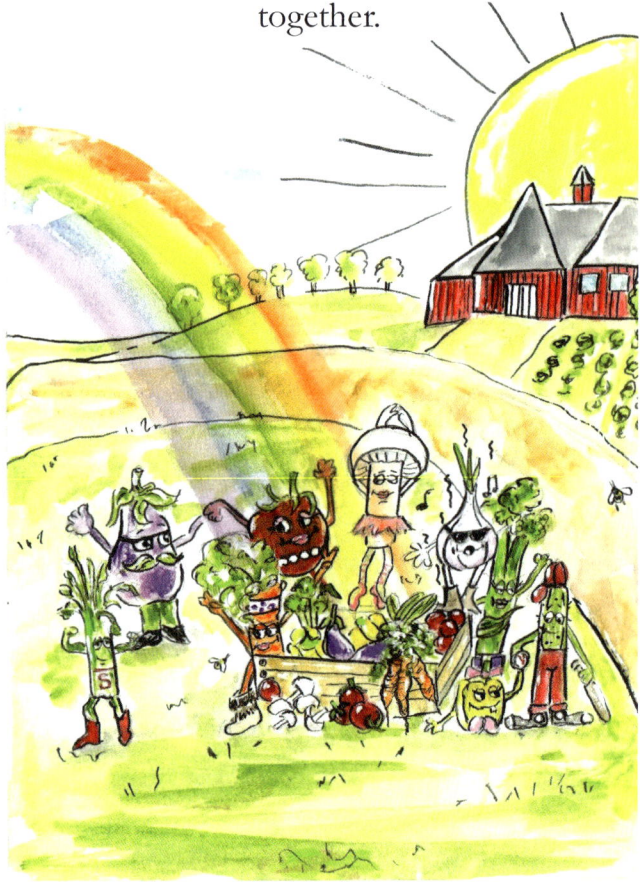

This book is for all kids who have
been told to eat their vegetables;
especially Brittany and Madilyn. I
love you both to the moon and
back!
Mom

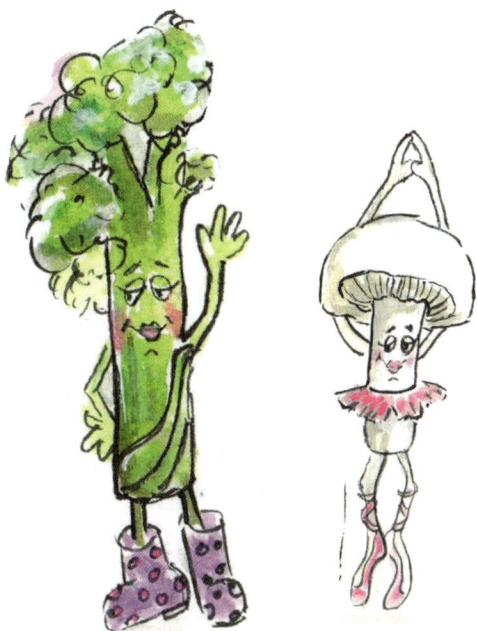

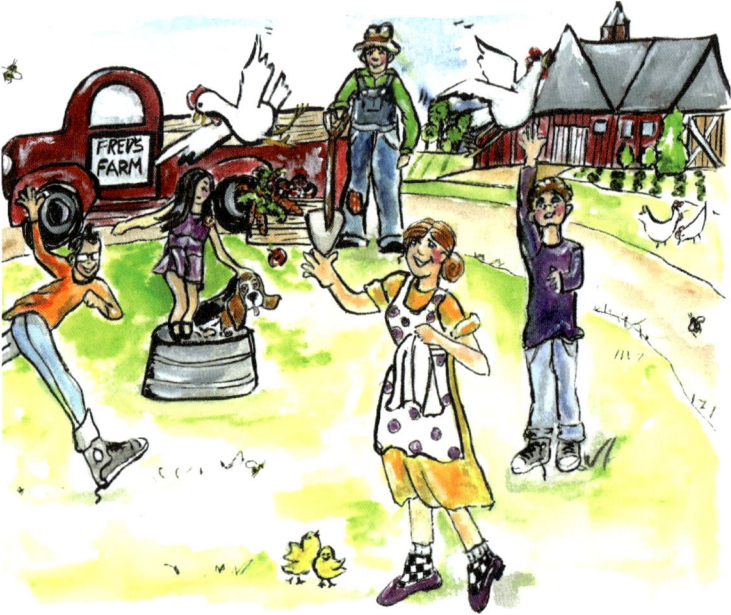

Farmer Fred lived on a beautiful
farm in the Country with his wife,
Mary, and their three children. They
grew fruits and vegetables of all
shapes, sizes, and colors and sold them
to a big grocery store in the city.

Every day Farmer Fred would load
up his truck with all his wonderful
fruits and vegetables and go into the
city, so there were plenty of fruits and
vegetables to feed all the families living
there. He always returned home in the
evening with an empty truck ready to
be filled up for the next day.

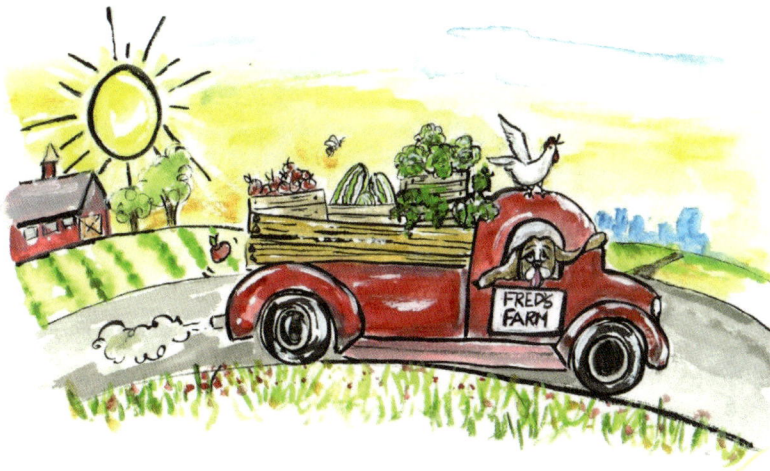

There was another family who lived on the farm, a vegetable family, The Sunny's. The vegetable family included Edgar Eggplant, he was the Dad and was a beautiful shade of purple. The Mom, Tammy, who was a gorgeous red tomato and their seven children.

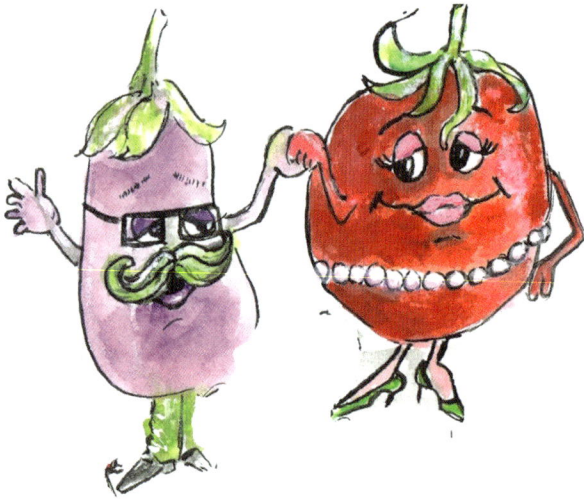

Their children were, Christopher Cucumber, Brittany Broccoli and Sammy Spinach; who were all wonderful shades of green. Carolyn Carrot who was bright orange. Madilyn Mushroom and George Garlic who were pure white. And the baby of the family, Yazmine the sunshine yellow pepper.

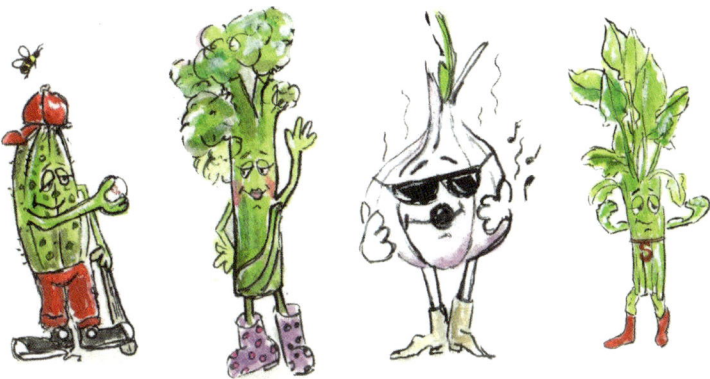

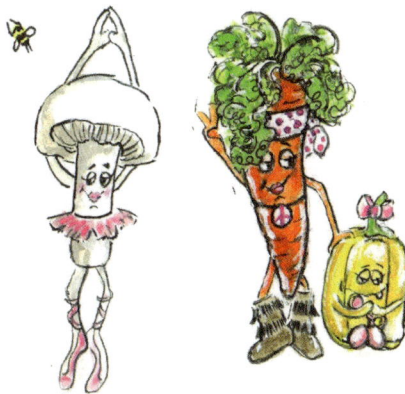

Early one morning, Farmer Fred loaded up all the vegetables into his truck for the delivery into the city. But this trip was different than all the others. Instead of coming home with an empty truck, Farmer Fred came home with his truck full of all the fruits and vegetables. The grocery store in the city didn't need the vegetables. They said no one was buying them.

"Why wasn't anyone buying fruits and vegetables" wondered Farmer Fred. "If no one wants our vegetables, we'll have to close the farm." Farmer Fred and Mary didn't know what to do.

When the Sunny Family heard no one was buying vegetables they had to do something about it. They couldn't lose the Farm they loved so dearly!! But what could they do?? They were just colorful vegetables.

As the Sunny family looked around the farm they saw Farmer Fred's kids playing outdoors in the sunshine. They were riding their bikes, playing games, running and jumping in the grass. They were so happy. But isn't this how all kids are? The Sunny family started to think about all the beautiful different colored fruits and vegetables Farmer Fred's family ate at every meal. They ate a rainbow of colors all the time. This MUST be why they were so happy the Sunny family thought. But if Farmer Fred's kids on the farm were so happy because they played outside and ate beautiful fruits and vegetables with every meal, what could the city kids be eating if no one was buying the fruits and vegetables anymore?

The next day Farmer Fred went into
the city to try and sell his colorful
fruits and vegetables again. The
Sunny family decided to go along
for the ride and do some investigat-
ing for themselves.

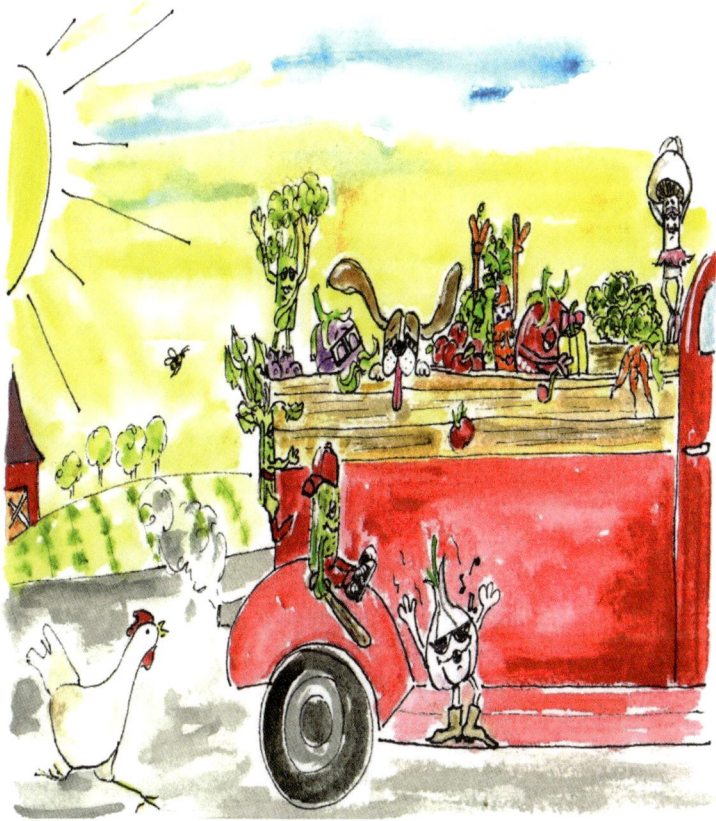

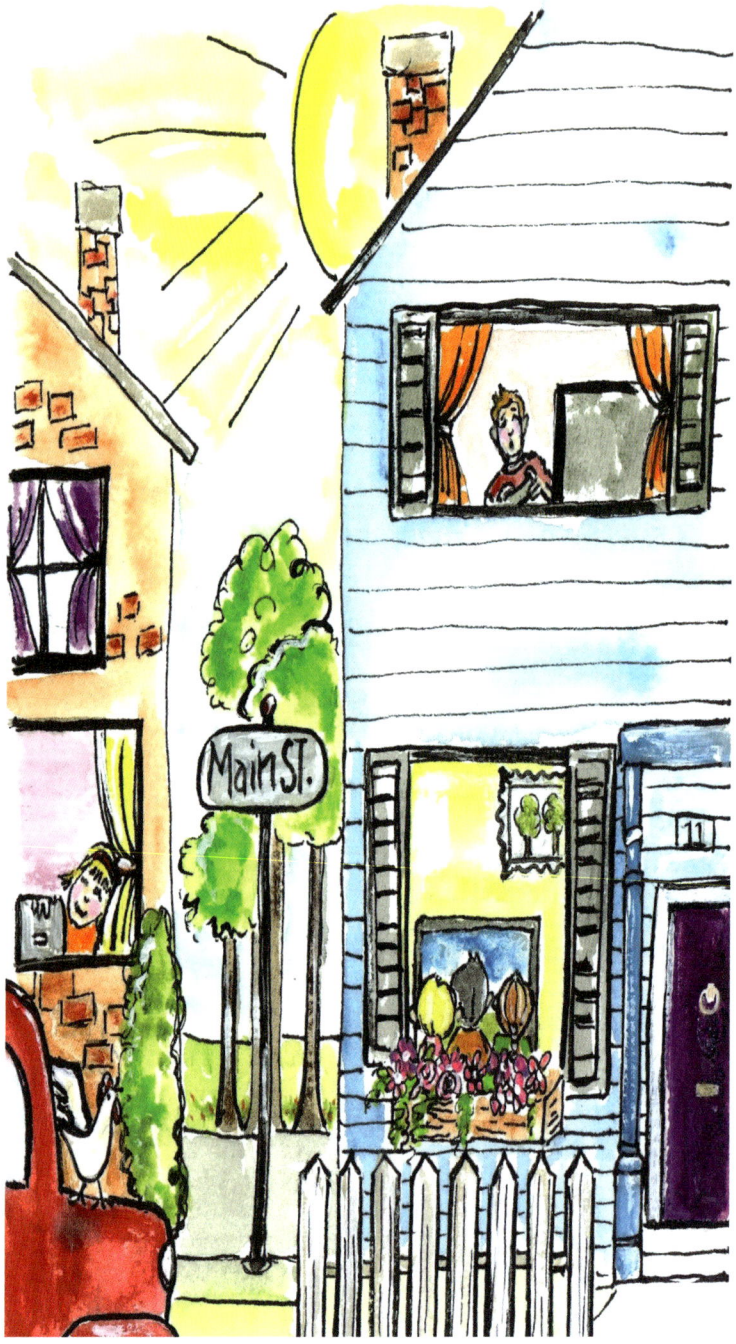

When the Sunny family got to the city
they couldn't believe what they saw.
Kids weren't outside playing in the sunshine and fresh air.   There were no kids
outside riding their bikes or running
and playing.
Where could they all be?
Then the Sunny family realized all the
kids were in their houses staring at
screens. They were watching TV, playing video games or looking at tablets
and cell phones. But, what exactly were
they looking at?

Lots and lots of colors, on everything; all the games they were playing were filled with colors and the TV shows were all colorful too. But, these children didn't look as happy as Farmer Fred's kids, who spent their days outside running and playing.

Then the Sunny Family noticed something else, the city kids weren't eating beautiful colorful meals with fruits and vegetables like Farmer Fred's kids ate.

The kids in the city all ate the same bland color, chicken nuggets and French fries, grilled cheese, macaroni and cheese, chips and soda. These foods are ok to eat sometimes, but maybe the city kids didn't know how good fruits and vegetables could taste and what all the beautiful colors could do for their health.

How could the Sunny family show them that they needed to eat as many colors as they were watching all day? By eating more colors, they would feel better, sleep better, be able to concentrate more at school, and have more energy. As the Sunny family was thinking about a way to teach the kids about eating more fruits and vegetables they noticed a big storm coming in.

The sky got dark. It got very windy and it started to thunder, lightning and rain. Suddenly a bolt of lightning hit the main transformer in the city where all the houses get their electricity. The entire city went dark!!

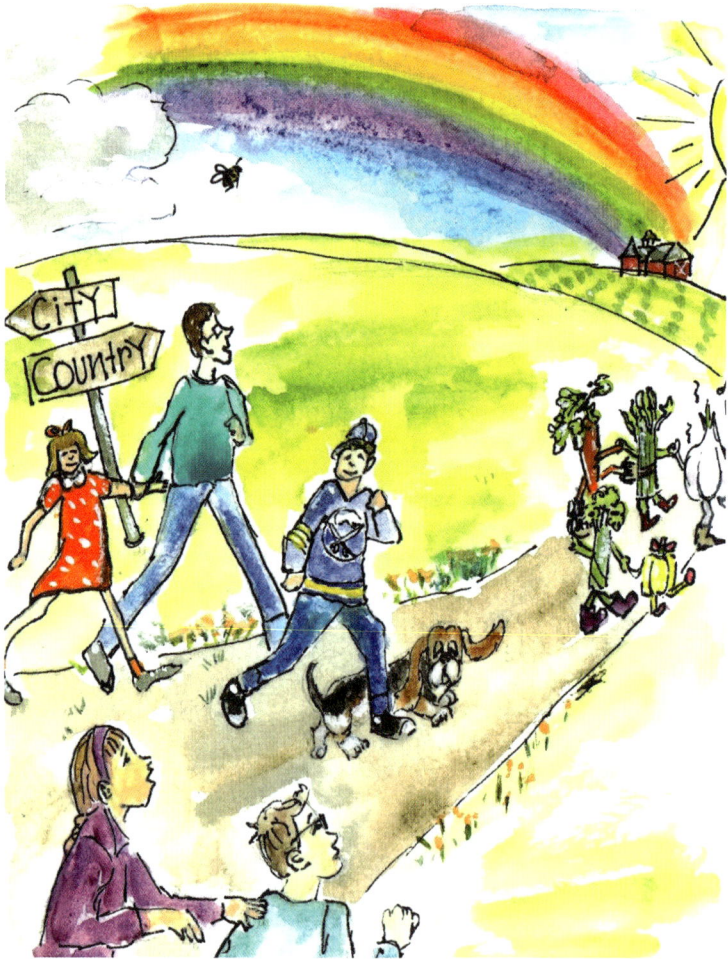

When the storm passed, everyone came out of their houses, almost like zombies. No one in the city had electricity, it was going to take the workers a couple of days to fix the transformer and all the power lines. The Sunny Family knew this was their chance. They finally had everyone's attention.

As the sun started to come back out it created a giant beautiful colorful rainbow that stretched from the city to the farm. The vegetables started following the colorful rainbow and hoped all the people in the city would follow along. They did!!!

The Sunny family decided to put on a show to teach the kids and their parents all the great things fruits and vegetables can do for their health.

As the families from the city got to the farm they saw all the beautiful fields of food growing. Farmer Fred's family greeted everyone and welcomed them to explore the farm. The entire Sunny family was busy getting set up on stage, ready to perform. The families all gathered around, excited to see the show.

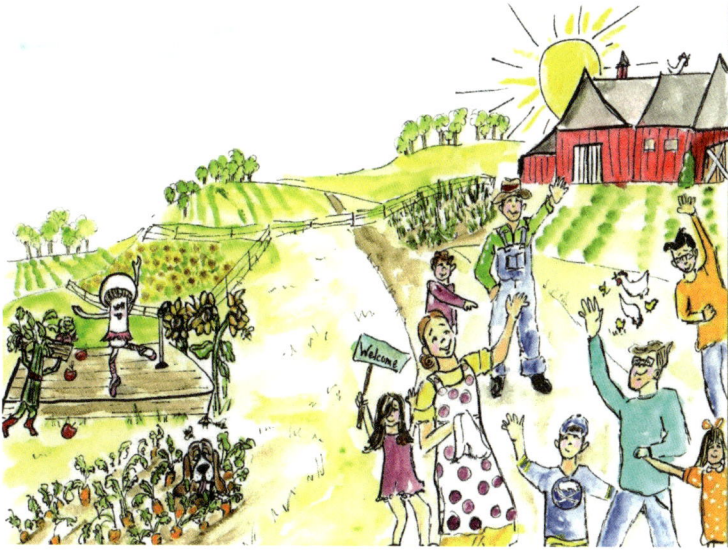

Edgar Eggplant took the stage. "Hello Everyone," Edgar said, "my name is Edgar and I'm an Eggplant. Today my family and I are going to talk to you about many different colored fruits and vegetables you see in the supermarket, and what all those colors can do for your health. Most people don't realize just how much what they eat can affect how they feel.

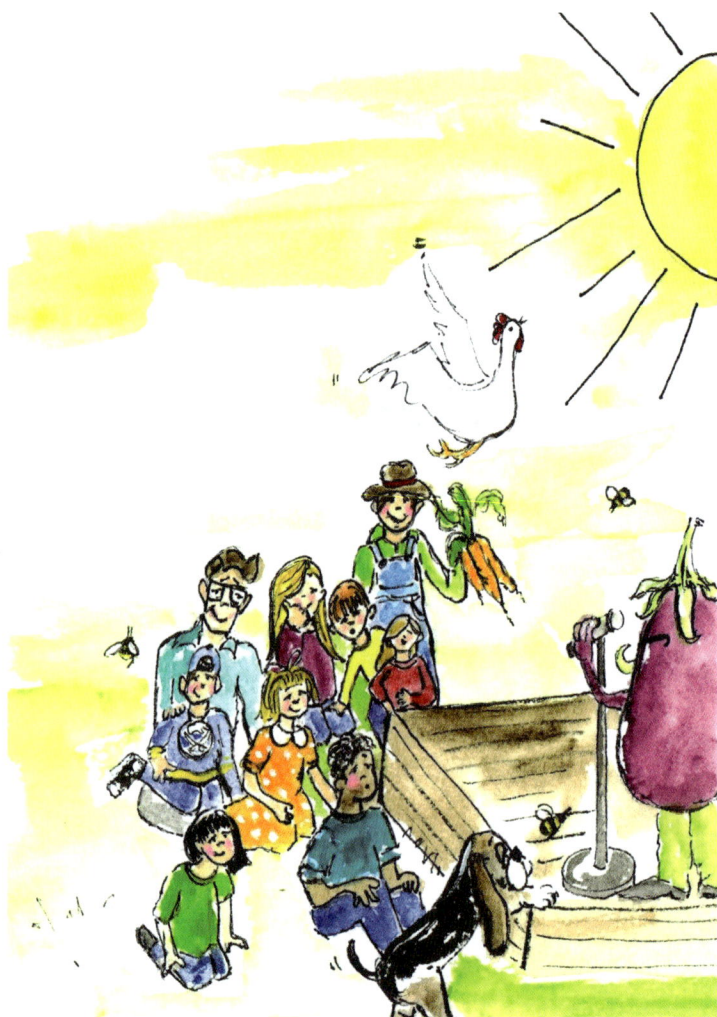

So, let's get started and bring out some of my family and friends". Joining him on stage was his brother, Barry the Blueberry, and his cousins Patty Plum, Betty Beet and Robert Raspberry. These fruits and vegetables are beautiful shades of blues and purples. Edgar asked the crowd, "do you know what eating blue and purple fruits and vegetables do for you?" Edgar went on to tell everyone that blue and purple foods help our brains!! These foods can make us smarter and they help keep us looking young. The families from the city had no idea these beautiful colored fruits and vegetables did things for their brains. People in the audience started whispering to each other, "maybe we need to eat more blue and purple foods to help our brains".

Next out came our green friends. Christopher the Cucumber, Brittany Broccoli, Sammy Spinach with their friend Laurie Lettuce. Green fruits and vegetables are good for all parts of your body. The darker the green the better!! They contain vitamins A, C and K. Vitamin A helps your eyes and bones; including your teeth. Vitamin C helps you grow big and strong.

Your body doesn't make or store vitamin C on its own, so it's important to include plenty of fruits and vegetables every day that contain vitamin C.

Vitamin K helps your blood. When you fall and get a scrap or bruise, vitamin K helps to heal those wounds. Some green vegetables are a good source of iron too, which also helps your blood. "Wow", thought the City families, "what we eat helps our bones, teeth and blood????"

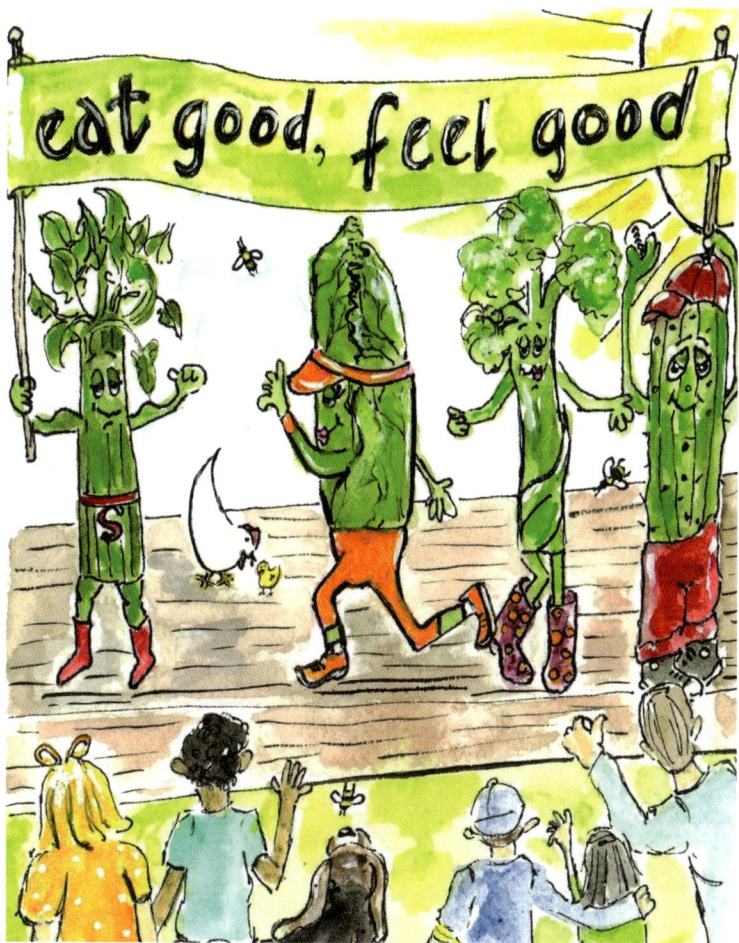

"Let's bring out our white fruits and vegetables. Madilyn the Mushroom, George
Garlic along with their friends Barbara the
Banana, Peggy Potato and Olly Onion."
What do white foods do for you? White
foods are high in potassium and fiber.
These foods protect your cells from dam-
age and may help lower our risk for cer-
tain diseases. This means as you get older,
less trips to the doctor! What you eat
helps your cells too?? This is incredible!

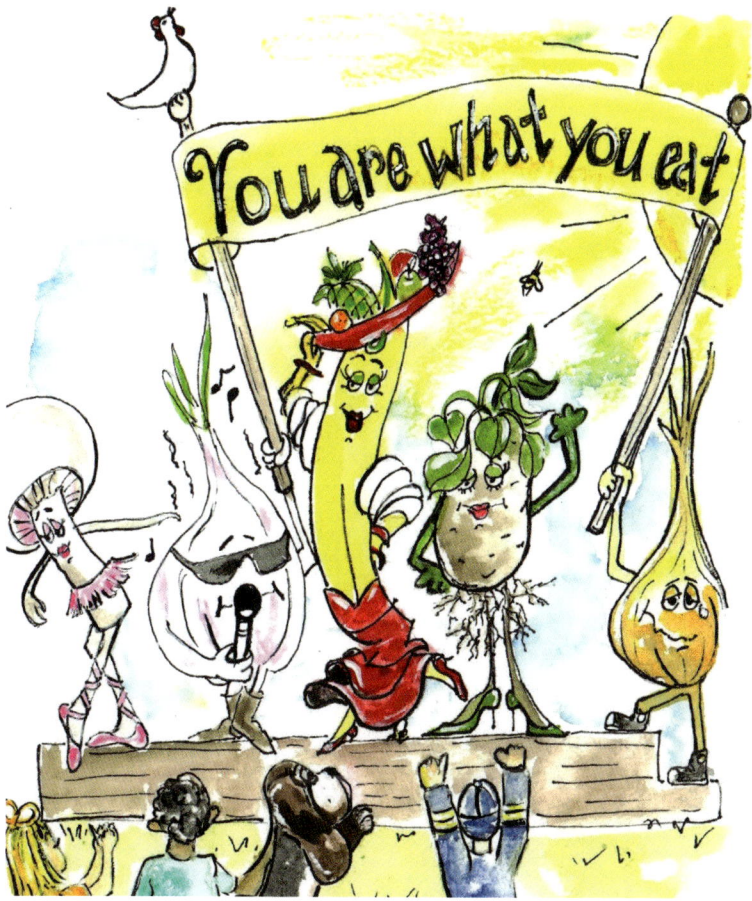

"Say hello to our Yellow and Orange friends!!!" The baby of the family, Yazmine the Yellow Pepper leading the way, with her is her Aunt Paula the Pineapple and her kids. Paula's daughter and son, Sally Squash and Peter Pear.

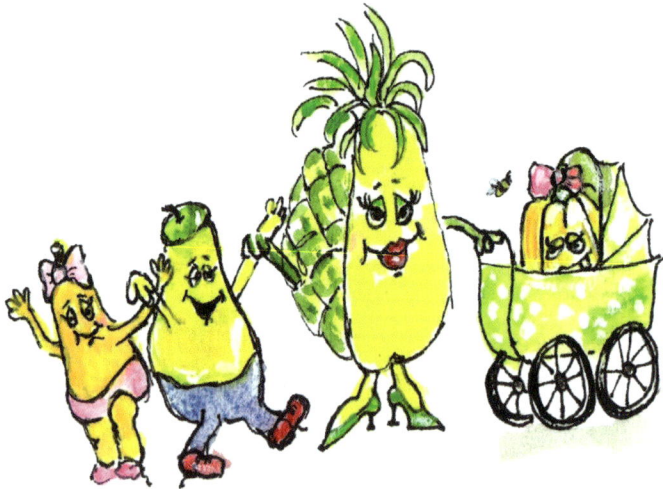

They were joined by their orange friends, Carolyn Carrot along with Oliver Orange and Amber Apricot. Yellow and Orange fruits and vegetables are loaded with Vitamin C and helps to protect you from getting sick. They also help you have nice skin and hair. Orange foods are great for your bones and teeth, just like their green friends.

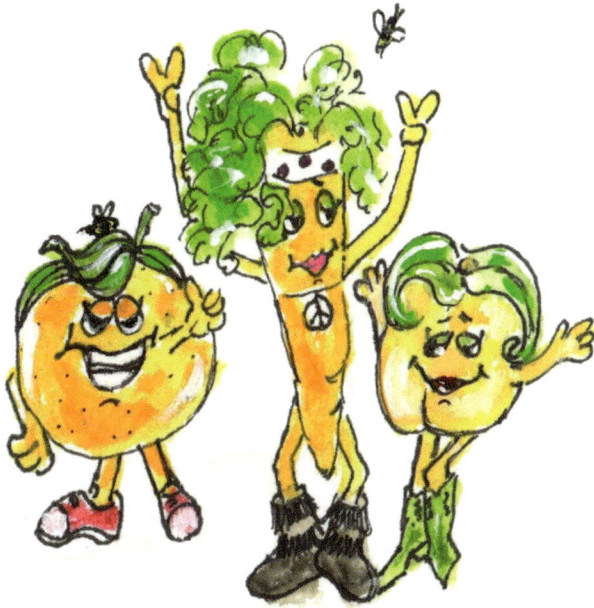

Last, we have our radiant reds! Out came Mama, Tammy the Tomato also with her is her sister Susie Strawberry and brother Charlie Cherry. Red fruits and vegetables, like the others we discussed, are high in Vitamins A and C to help prevent you from getting sick. Red foods are also great for your eyes, heart and help with memory. Bet you could use a lot of Red Vegetables while you're in school. Think of how helpful they could be to you during Math or Spelling lessons.

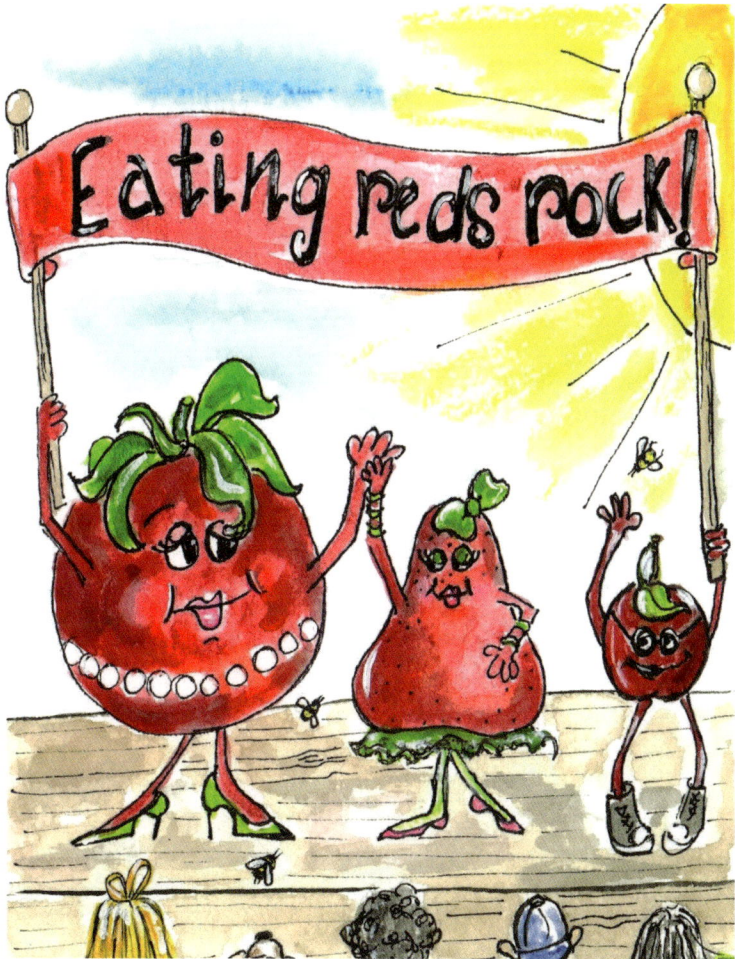

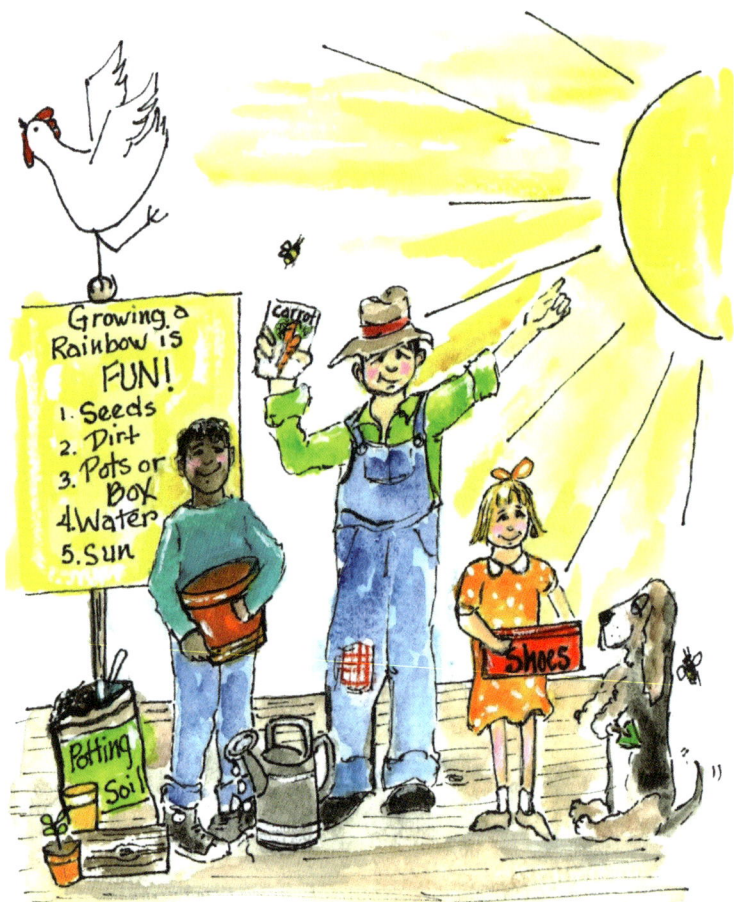

Growing a
Rainbow is
FUN!
1. Seeds
2. Dirt
3. Pots or
   Box
4. Water
5. Sun

Carrot

Potting
Soil

Shoes

Farmer Fred hopped up on stage and showed the kids that growing your own fruits and vegetables can be fun. You don't need a big garden, you can grow vegetables anywhere, in a pot, in a box, even in a shoe! Just pick your favorite seeds and get some dirt. Just like you, plants need plenty of sunshine and water. So, make sure your plant is in a sunny spot, give it water every day and soon you'll have your own vegetables.

Helping your parents cook can also be fun, ask your Mom or Dad if you can help with dinner some night. Maybe they'll let you go to the grocery store with them and pick a fruit or vegetable you've never tried before. There are so many options available, I'm sure you'll find one you LOVE!

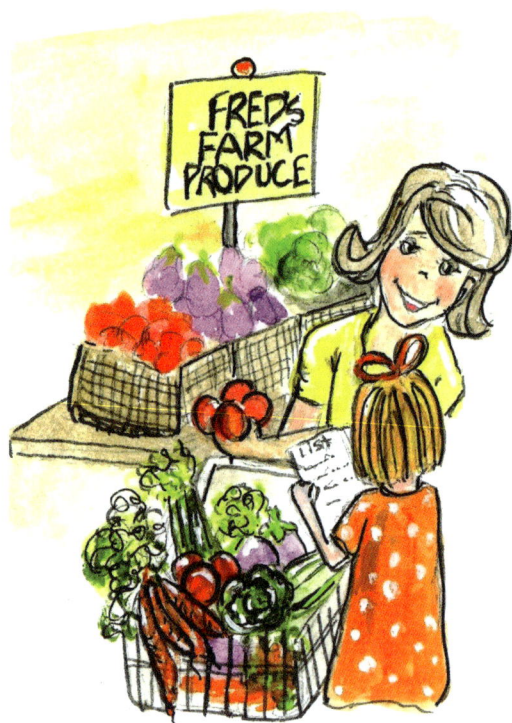

The city kids had no idea how great all the different colored fruits and vegetables were for them. Eating different colored fruits and vegetables help you not get sick as often, they are good for your bones, teeth and all the cells in your body. What you eat also affects your brain and your mind, even your hair and skin.

They learned that there are many different fruits and vegetables and what all the colors could do for them! The City kids cheered!! They were so happy to learn about all the great vitamins and nutrients in the different colors of fruits and vegetables. They now know that it's important to eat a rainbow of colors and try to have one fruit and one vegetable with EVERY meal.

They all went back to the city knowing that when they saw Farmer Fred's truck at the grocery store every day that there would be new fruits and vegetables for them to try which will help them feel better and have more energy. All the vitamins and nutrients in the fruits and vegetables will mean they'll spend less time sick, concentrate better, and do well in school. Plus, they'll have more energy to have fun and play after school.

Being outside in the sun and fresh air provides your body with nutrients and vitamins too. Eating right and staying active will ensure you grow up strong, happy and healthy. When you look at your plate at meals, look for the rainbow!!

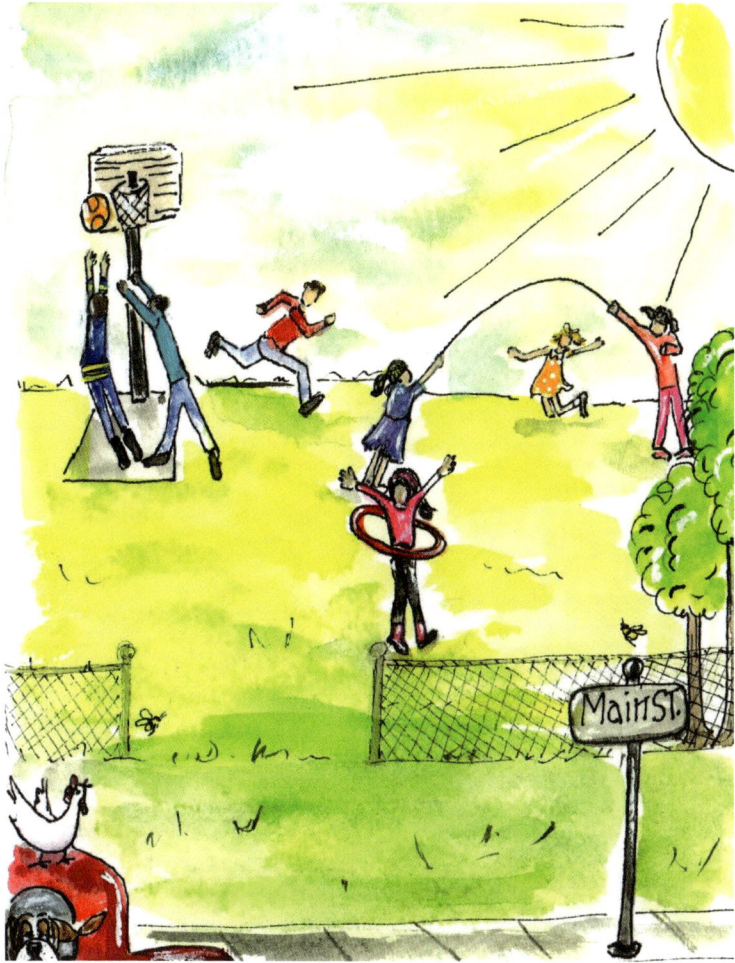

Still not so sure if you like fruits and vegetables? A great way to get lots of fruits and vegetables in a meal is to have a smoothie. You can even put vegetables in smoothies and there are so many different colors and flavors you can try.

Try this recipe that includes all the colors of the rainbow:

1 cup of frozen strawberries

1 frozen banana

1 cup of spinach leaves

1 cup of frozen blueberries

1 cup of frozen pineapple

2-3 cups of orange juice (enough liquid so your blender doesn't work too hard and gives a good smooth consistency).

Add all of the above ingredients to a blender and blend until smooth. If needed add additional orange juice to get a nice smooth creamy consistency. Then enjoy! You can add any fruit or vegetable you'd like, try substituting different colored fruits and/or vegetables. See what you like best.

ABOUT THE AUTHOR

Shari Fruchtel is a Certified Holistic Health and Nutrition Coach and mother of two daughters. She trained at the Institute for Integrative Nutrition on over 100 different diet theories and how they affect Health and Wellness. Shari is also the owner and founder of SHARIng Health with Shari and resides in Buffalo New York. I was lead to Health Coaching while navigating through my own health issues and decided there is too much confusing information, too many fad diets and miracle solutions in the media today. I realized from that moment on that I had a passion for Health, Nutrition and Wellness and started my journey, and haven't slowed down since. I want to share my knowledge of Health and Wellness with everyone especially children. Children's Health and Nutrition are VERY important to me. Sharing with all children and hoping to give them the tools to live a Healthy, Happy lifestyle are my mission. Make it a Happy Healthy Day!

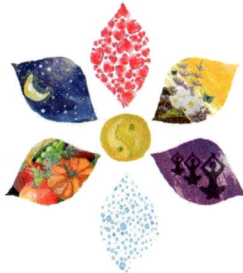

SHARIng Health
with Shari

65211452R00023

Made in the USA
Charleston, SC
14 December 2016